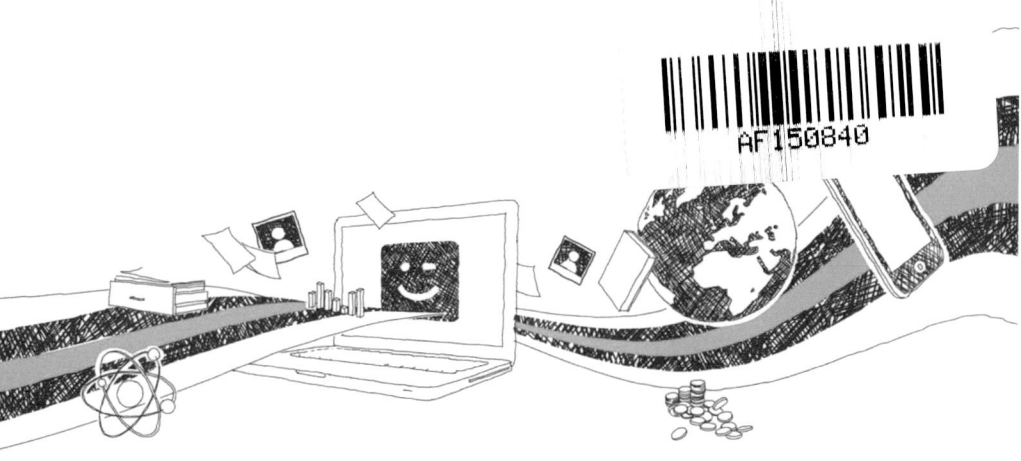
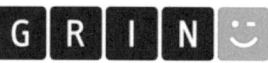

Bibliographic information published by the German National Library:

The German National Library lists this publication in the National Bibliography;
detailed bibliographic data are available on the Internet at http://dnb.dnb.de .

Imprint:

Copyright © 2016 GRIN Verlag, Open Publishing GmbH
Print and binding: Books on Demand GmbH, Norderstedt Germany
ISBN: 9783668257870

This book at GRIN:

http://www.grin.com/en/e-book/335626/effect-of-dried-blood-rumen-content-
mixture-dbrcm-on-feed-intake-body

M. B. Yitbarek, B. T. Mersso, A. M. Wosen

Effect of Dried Blood-Rumen Content Mixture (DBRCM) on feed intake, body weight gain, feed conversion ratio and mortality rate of SASSO C44 broiler chicks

GRIN Publishing

GRIN - Your knowledge has value

Since its foundation in 1998, GRIN has specialized in publishing academic texts by students, college teachers and other academics as e-book and printed book. The website www.grin.com is an ideal platform for presenting term papers, final papers, scientific essays, dissertations and specialist books.

Visit us on the internet:

http://www.grin.com/

http://www.facebook.com/grincom

http://www.twitter.com/grin_com

Effect of Dried Blood-Rumen Content Mixture (DBRCM) on feed intake, body weight gain, feed conversion ratio and mortality rate of SASSO C44 broiler chicks

M.B. Yitbarek[1*], B.T. Mersso [2], A.M. Wosen[2]

[1]Department of Animal Science, College of Agriculture and Natural Resources, Debre Markos University, Debre Markos, [2] Department of Animal Production Studies, College of Veterinary Medicine and Agriculture, Addis Ababa University, Addis Ababa, Ethiopia

Received on 10/5/2016; Accepted on 25/5/2016

Abstract

The objective of this experiment was to determine the effect of dried blood- rumen content mixtures (DBRCM) on the performance of SASSO C44 broiler chicks. A total of 225 unsexed day old broiler chicks (SASSO C44) were randomly distributed to five dietary treatment groups in a completely randomized design and replicated thrice with 15 birds per replicate. The experimental diets were formulated to contain 100%Soyabean meal(SBM)+0%DBRCM (T1), 80%SBM+20% DBRCM (T2),60%SBM+ 40% DBRCM (T3), 40%SBM+60% DBRCM(T4) and 20%SBM+80% DBRCM (T5) in 56 days of age. Both starter and finisher diets were formulated to be iso-caloric and iso-nitrogenous. Data were collected on average feed intake, body weight gain (BWG), feed conversion ratio (FCR) and mortality rate. The result revealed that the daily dry matter intake was ranged from 75.8 to 80.4g/day/bird in the entire experimental period of growth. Birds fed on T5 (75.8) was lower (P<0.05) DMI compared with T1 (79.0g), T2 (78.9g), T3 (80.4g). The mean daily body weight gain of birds ranged from 26.4g to 31.6g and no marked significant difference (P>0.05) among each treatment groups. The feed conversion ratio(FCR) ranged from 2.5-2.9 and there was no statistical marked difference (P>0.05) among treatment groups. Also there was no statistical difference (P>0.05) in mortality rate. Based on the present result, it could be concluded that dried blood rumen content mixture can be included up to 60% inclusion level for starter phases and up to 80% for finisher phases of growth to replace soybean meal without any adverse effect on bodyweight gain, FCR, and mortality rate of birds.

Keywords: body weight gain; DBRCM; FCR; mortality rate; broiler chick; Ethiopia.

Introduction

Bovine blood-rumen content mixture (BBRCM) is an abattoir (slaughter house) by-product that offers a tremendous potential as a cheap and locally available alternative feedstuff for poultry (Adeniji and Jimoh, 2007). The same source indicated that BBRCM has a little or no cost and can be incorporated in poultry rations after appropriate processing in order to reduce production costs and alleviate pollution problems without any reported deleterious clinical effects on animal health and their performance. Abattoirs generate large amounts of solid waste and effluents such as rumen contents, blood and wash water. According to CSA (2013) cattle population in Ethiopia is 53.99 million. By considering an off-take rate of 7% for cattle (Bisrat, 2013) around 3.8 million cattle is slaughtered annually, and a recovery rate of 2.7-3.5 kg (DM basis) of ruminal contents (Dominguez et al., 1994) and 3-4% of its body weight blood per head of a slaughtered animal produced (Liu, 2009). Approximately about 133000 quintal of DM rumen content and 38 million litres of blood per annum can be produced. In the separation into plasma and blood cell fractions, 60% plasma with a solids content of 8% and 40% corpuscles with a solids content of 38% is obtained. Therefore from 100 kg of blood, 4.8 kg of plasma powder and 15.2 kg corpuscle powder would be produced (Downes et al., 1987). Based on this calculation from 38 million litres of blood, 76000 quintal blood meal can be produced annually in Ethiopia. If a quintal of dried rumen content and blood meal is sold by 300 and 800 Ethiopian Birr respectively, 39.9 million Birr from dried rumen content and 60.8 million Birr from blood meal can be obtained. Therefore, without any use of this waste, Ethiopia has lost 100.6 million Birr annually. Similarly in Debre Markos, 5000 cattle are slaughtered formally in a municipal slaughter house per annum. Accordingly, an estimated 17500 kg DM rumen content and 50000 litres of blood (10000 kg blood meal) can be produced annually (calculated by considering 1 cattle- 250 kg body weight).

These huge amounts of rumen content and blood are not utilized for animal feeding, but simply released into the environment and difficulties in disposal of such wastes. The existing system of disposing abattoir wastes is resulting in pollution not only causing problems related to odour, flies and hygiene, but surface and ground water can be polluted with pathogens and undesirable chemical compounds. Efforts have not been made yet in Ethiopia in general and in Debre-Markos in particular to utilize these waste products as an alternative feed ingredient in broiler rations.

The need to maximize the economic benefits and minimize the disposal problems associated with rumen content and blood, led to new interests in the investigation of these by-products for a possible use in the diets of broilers as a feed ingredient and source of protein that can replace soybean meal, an expensive feed ingredient for poultry rations in Ethiopia. Therefore, this study was conducted to evaluate the performance of broilers fed diets containing dried bovine blood-rumen content mixtures as replacement for soybean meal.

Materials and methods

The study area

The study was conducted in Debre-Markos, Ethiopia. Debre-Markos is located at 300 km from Addis Ababa in Northwest of the country and 265 km Southeast of Bahir Dar, capital of Amhara region. The mean altitude is 2400 meter above sea level. The annual rainfall ranges from 900-1800 mm and a minimum and maximum temperature of the area is $7.5^{O}C$ and $25^{O}C$, respectively.

Collecting and processing of blood

Fresh blood was collected from slaughtering house immediately after the cattle is slaughtered and boiled to $100^{O}C$ for 45 minutes in order to let water evaporate and destroy pathogenic organisms. The coagulate after boiling was spread on a clean plastic sheet over the spreading table to avoid any contamination on the ground and dried for 3-5 days, depending on weather condition, the amount of the materials spread and frequency of turning.

Collecting and processing of rumen content

Fresh rumen content obtained from freshly eviscerated cattle was collected into clean containers from Debre-Markos municipality slaughtering house. The rumen was split with the aid of a sharp knife and the contents emptied into a big metal vat. The metal vat containing the rumen content was placed on burning firewood and boiled for 2 hours with intermittent stirring to prevent burning until the mixture is almost free of steam. This was done to reduce the microbial load of the rumen content. The boiled rumen content was spread on a clean plastic sheet for sun drying. While drying, it was stirred and turned more than four times daily so as to facilitate even drying.

Mixing of dried blood and dried rumen content

Then dried blood and rumen content was mixed at 1:1 ratio to produce dried blood-rumen content mixture that was used to replace soybean meal at varied levels in rations of starter and finisher phases of growth.

Experimental Birds and their Management

Two hundred and twenty five day old unsexed SASSO C44 broiler chicks were purchased from Mekelle poultry farms PLC. All the chicks were randomly allocated to the pens, using a Completely Randomized Design (CRD). The experimental rooms were divided into fifteen separate pens (0.12 m^2 /bird) of equal size 1.8 m^2 by using timber and mesh wire. The house was electrically heated using 200 watt bulbs per pen. The brooder temperature was maintained at about 32-35 °C for the first 7 days of age and monitor frequently for about 3 times per day (in the morning, during the day, and at night). Clean and disinfected feeder and waterer were provided in each pen. Standard vaccination schedule was done and strict sanitary measures were followed during the experimental period. The experimental ration, containing dried blood rumen content mixture as replacement of soybean meal was formulated and fed for 56 days of experimental period.

Treatments and experimental rations

All broiler chicks were individually weighed and randomly allocated to five dietary treatments replicated thrice with fifteen birds per replicate in a completely randomized design (CRD). The feed ingredients used in formulation of different experimental rations for the study were maize (*Zea mays*), wheat middling, noug seedcake (*Guizotia abyssinica*), roasted soybean (*Glysine max*), vitamin premix, lysine, methionine, salt and limestone.

The test diets for the starter phase (1-28 days) were formulated to be isocaloric and isonitrogenous containing 3000 kcal ME /kg DM and 23% CP, and the finisher phase (29-56 days) contain 3200 kcal ME/kg and 20 % CP to meet the requirements of starter and finisher phases of broiler (NRC,1994).

Rations were formulated based on the results of the chemical analysis of the feed ingredients, and the control diet was formulated to contain about 30% soybean meals from the total ration. Therefore, based on 30% soybean meals, the treatments contained in T1 (100% Soybean roasted+0% DBRCM), T2 (80% Soybean roasted+20% DBRCM), T3 (60% Soybean roasted+40% DBRCM), T4 (40% Soybean roasted+60% DBRCM) and T5 (20% Soybean roasted+80% DBRCM).

Measurements

Average dry matter intake (ADMI), body weight gain, feed conversion ratio and mortality percentage were recorded to evaluate the difference between the treatment rations. Feed and water were provided ad-libitum. Feed offered and refusals were weighed and recorded every day (g/day) throughout the experimental period to estimate the feed intake for each replicate and treatment. Feed intake was determined by difference from the quantity offered and refused daily. Dry matter and nutrient intakes were calculated by difference from offered and refusals on dry matter basis. The live weights of birds were weighed individually from each replicate at the beginning of the experiment and weekly till the end of the experiment. Body weight gain was calculated as a difference between two consequent weighing of body weight, and average daily weight gain (ADG) was calculated as body weight change divided by the number of experimental days. Feed conversion ratio was calculated as unit weight of feed consumed per unit body weight change. Nutrient conversion ratio (CP, MEI, CF and Ca) was also calculated by dividing the nutrient intake to body weight gain. Daily mortality was recorded for each replicate and treatment, and then weekly mortality rate was calculated by subtracting the number of dead chicks from the number of live chicks at each interval.

Chemical Analysis

Representative samples were taken from each of the feed ingredients used in the experiment to National Veterinary Institute at Bishofitu, Ethiopia for chemical analysis and analyzed before formulating the actual dietary treatments. In the same way, samples were taken from each of the treatment diets at each mixing and from refusals every day during the experiment and kept in paper bags until analyzed. The refusal from each pen was collected each morning before fresh feed is given, cleaned from external contaminants by use of 5 mm mesh size sieve and by hand picking, weighed and pooled by treatment, thoroughly mixed and sample was taken and the rest discarded. All samples were analyzed for dry matter (DM), ether extract (EE), crude fiber (CF) and ash (A.O.A.C., 2000). Nitrogen was determined by kjeldhal procedure and CP was calculated by multiplying N content by 6.25. Calcium was determined by atomic absorption spectrometer after dry ashing. The Metabolizable energy (ME) levels of feed ingredients was calculated using the formula ME (Kcal/kg DM) = 3951 + 54.4 EE - 88.7 CF - 40.8 Ash (Wiseman, 1987).

Statistical analysis

The experiment was arranged in completely randomized design (CRD). All collected data was subjected to analysis of variance (ANOVA) using the general linear models procedure by SAS (Version 9.2) software and for crosschecking, SPSS (Version.20) software was employed. When treatment effects were found to be significant (P<0.05), mean separation was undertaken using Turkey HSD test. All values were calculated on a pen average basis.

Results

The blood and rumen content were collected immediately after the animal was slaughtered and processed separately, and then mixed a 1:1 ratio to make dried blood rumen content mixture (DBRCM). The blood meal, dried rumen content and DBRCM were taken for chemical analysis to National Veterinary Institute (NVI), Bishofitu, Ethiopia. The chemical composition of blood meal, dried rumen content and DBRCM were presented in Table 1. The chemical composition of feed ingredients used for experimental diets is presented in Table 2.

Table 1. Chemical composition of blood meal, dried rumen content and dried blood- rumen content mixtures (DBRCM) collected and processed in Debre Markos as DM basis.

No	Feed type	DM	MM	CF	CP	EE	Ca	NFE	Kcal ME/Kg DM
1	Blood Meal	94	4.36	2.87	83.5	0.64	1.42	2.63	3553.359
2	DRC	93.1	11.28	31.79	16.2	2.02	1.79	31.81	780.891
3	DBRCM	93.3	7.5	15.75	36.93	1.48	1.43	31.64	2328.487

DRC- Dried Rumen Content; DBRCM- Dried Blood Rumen Content Mixture; DM -Dry Matter; CP-Crude Protein; ME-Metabolizable Energy; CF-Crude Fiber; EE-Ether Extract; MM-Mineral Matter NFE-Nitrogen Free Extract; Ca-Calcium.

Table 2. Chemical composition of feed ingredients used for preparing experimental diets as DM basis

No	Feed type	DM	MM	CF	CP	EE	Ca	NFE	Kcal ME/Kg DM
1	DBRCM	93.3	7.5	15.75	36.93	1.48	1.43	31.64	2328.487
2	NSC	94.6	8.88	23.35	38.46	7.27	2.47	16.64	1913.039
3	Maize (White)	90.7	0.63	1.65	7.45	4.98	1.29	75.99	4049.853
4	Soybean/Roasted/	96.8	5.65	14.77	32.17	13.29	2.07	30.92	3133.357
5	Wheat Middling	90.3	3.06	6.53	17.72	4.21	1.66	58.78	3475.965

DBRCM- Dried Blood Rumen Content Mixture; NSC- Noug Seed Cake; DM -Dry Matter; CP-Crude Protein; ME-Metabolizable Energy; CF-Crude Fiber; EE-Ether Extract; MM-Mineral Matter NFE-Nitrogen Free Extract; Ca-Calcium.

Feed ingredients of starter and finisher ration

The feed ingredients and chemical composition of the five dietary treatment groups of starter and finisher ration is presented in Table 3.

Dry matter and nutrient intake during the starter phase

Mean daily nutrient intake of SASSO C44 broiler chicks (1-28 days) fed different level of dried blood rumen content mixture as a replacement for soybean meal is presented in Table 4. The average daily dry mater intake of birds was 40.4, 39.9, 40.3, 38.6 and 38.5for T1, T2, T3, T4 and T5, respectively. There was no statistically marked significant difference (P>0.05) in daily DMI among treatment groups. However birds fed on T1 (0% DBRCM) were higher (P<0.05) total DMI than T5 (80%DBRCM). Birds fed on T2 (20%DBRCM) had higher (P<0.05) daily CPI compared with T5 (80%DBRCM). Birds fed on T5 (1.5g) had lower (P<0.05) CFI compared with T1 (0%DBRCM) and T3 (40%DBRCM). There was no significant difference (P>0.05) in ME intake of birds among the treatment groups. Higher (P<0.05) Ca intake was observed on T3 and T4 than T2 and T5.

Dry matter and nutrient intake during the finisher phase

The mean dry matter and nutrient intake of birds during the finisher phase of growth is presented in Table 4. The mean daily DMI during the finisher phase in five dietary treatments were 116.2, 116.4, 119.1, and 116.9, 111.1gram/bird/day for T1, T2, T3, T4 and T5, respectively. T5 (111.1g) had the lowest (P<0.05) daily DMI compared with other treatments. Birds fed on T5 (80%DBRCM) had the lowest (P<0.05) total DM, CP, CF and Ca intake among other treatment groups. Birds fed on T5 (p<0.05) had lower MEI compared with T3.

Dry matter and nutrient intake of birds during the entire experiment

The mean dry matter and nutrient intake of birds during the entire experiment is presented in Table 4. The daily DMI of birds fed on the dietary treatments were 79.0, 78.9, 80.4, 78.5 and 75.8 gram for T1, T2, T3, T4 and T5, respectively. Birds fed on T5 had the lowest DMI (p<0.05) compared with T1, T2 and T3, and birds fed on T5 (80%DBRCM) had shown the lowest (P<0.05) total dry matter intake (TDMI) compared with T1, T2, and T3.

Furthermore birds fed on T5 had the lowest (P<0.05) CP and CF intake compared with other treatment groups. There was a similar (P>0.05) MEI in all treatment groups in 56 days of age. The average Ca intake of a birds were on T3 and T4 >T1 and T2>T5 (P<0.05).

Body weight change during the starter phase

The body weight change of birds during the starter phase is presented in Table 5. Nearly similar body weight of broiler chicks were allocated in five dietary treatments during the starter phase of growth for 28 days.

The mean daily weight gains of birds were 26.1, 26.0, 24.6, 25.5 and 23.5g for T1, T2, T3, T4 and T5, respectively. Birds fed on T5 (80%DBRCM) had lower (P<0.05) mean daily body weight gain compared with T1 (0%DBRCM). T5 had lower (P<0.05) final body weight and mean total body weight gain compared with T1.

Table 3. Proportion of ingredients used in formulating broiler starter and finisher rations and chemical composition of the treatment groups

Ingredients in %	Starter ration					Finisher ration				
	T1	T2	T3	T4	T5	T1	T2	T3	T4	T5
SBM(Roasted)	30	24	18	12	6	30	24	18	12	6
DBRCM	0	6	12	18	24	0	6	12	18	24
Maize(White)	34.2	36.6	35.2	36.1	36.2	40.7	42.2	43.2	45.5	46.0
NSC	24.4	24.7	21.8	21.5	20.6	13.8	12.5	12.4	11.7	9.9
Wheat middling	8.8	6.1	10.4	9.8	10.6	12.7	12.7	11.8	10.2	11.5
Limestone	1.2	1.2	1.2	1.2	1.2	1.2	1.2	1.2	1.2	1.2
Vitamin premix	0.5	0.5	0.5	0.5	0.5	0.5	0.5	0.5	0.5	0.5
Salt	0.5	0.5	0.5	0.5	0.5	0.5	0.5	0.5	0.5	0.5
Lysine	0.2	0.2	0.2	0.2	0.2	0.2	0.2	0.2	0.2	0.2
Methionine	0.2	0.2	0.2	0.2	0.2	0.2	0.2	0.2	0.2	0.2
Total	100	100	100	100	100	100	100	100	100	100
DM (%)	90	90	91	90	92	90.4	90.3	90.1	90.6	90.2
CP (% DM)	23.1	23.2	23.1	23.2	23.3	20.2	20.1	20.3	20.2	20.1
ME(kcal/Kg DM)	3097.7	3058.5	3047.5	3009.1	2975.4	3293.7	3281.3	3240.3	3216.2	3198.9
CF (% DM)	5.2	5.1	5.4	5.3	5.1	6.4	6.2	6.1	6.3	6.2
MM (% DM)	8.5	8.6	8.4	8.3	8.5	9.3	9.6	9.5	9.3	9.4
EE (% DM)	5.4	5.2	5.3	5.1	5.4	5.6	5.5	5.4	5.3	5.2
NFE (% DM)	57.8	57.9	57.8	58.1	57.7	58.5	58.6	58.7	58.9	59.1
Ca (% DM)	1.2	1.2	1.1	1.3	1.4	1.2	0.84	0.82	0.86	0.85	0.81

NOTE:SBM=soybean meal; DBRCM=Dried Blood Rumen Content Mixture;NSC= Noug SeedCake; T1=0%DBRCM+100%SBM,T2=20% DBRCM+80%SBM; T3=40%DBRCM+60%SBM;T4=60%DBRCM+40%SBM;T5=80%DBRCM+20%SBM; DM=Dry Matter; CP=Crude Protein;ME=Metabolizable Energy; CF=Crude Fiber; EE=Ether Extract; MM=Mineral Matter NFE=Nitrogen Free Extract; Ca=Calcium. Vitamin premix = 25 kg Broiler premix contains, Vitamin A 1000 000 IU, Vitamin D3 200 000 IU. Vitamin E 1000 mg, Vitamin K3 225 mg, Vitamin B1 125 mg, Vitamin B2 500 mg, Vitamin B3 1375 mg, Vitamin B6 125mg, Vitamin B12 2 mg, Vitamin PP (niacin) 4, 000 mg, Folic Acid, 100 mg, choline chloride 37,500 mg, Calcium 29.7 %, Iron 0.4 %, Copper 0.05 %. Manganese 0.6 %, Zinc 0.7%, Iodine 0.01 % Selenium 0.004 %

Table 4. DM and Nutrient intake of SASSO C44 broiler chicks during starter phase (1-28 days), finisher phase (29-56 days) and enter experiment (1-56 days)

Parameters	Experimental Diets						
	T1	T2	T3	T4	T5	SEM	P-value
Starter Phase							
Mean daily DM intake (g/bird)	40.4	39.9	40.3	38.6	38.5	0.282	0.051
Mean total DM intake (g/bird)	1130.9[a]	1117.6[ab]	1128.6[ab]	1081.5[ab]	1076.6[b]	7.907	0.047
Mean daily CP intake(g/bird)	10.6[a]	10.7[a]	10.5[ab]	10.5[ab]	10.2[b]	0.062	0.040
Mean daily CF intake(g/bird)	2.2[a]	2.1[ab]	2.2[a]	2.0[ab]	1.5[b]	0.081	0.019
Mean daily ME intake(kcal/bird)	161.2[a]	174.4[a]	160.5[a]	157.9[a]	155.8[a]	3.173	0.434
Mean daily Ca intake(g/bird)	0.57[ab]	0.50[b]	0.60[a]	0.60[a]	0.50[b]	0.013	0.002
Finisher phase							
Mean daily DM intake (g/bird)	116.2[a]	116.4[a]	119.1[a]	116.9[a]	111.8[b]	0.680	0.001
Mean total DM intake (g/bird)	3253.4[a]	3259.6[a]	3333.7[a]	3272.6[a]	3130.7[b]	19.093	0.001
Mean daily CP intake(g/bird)	26.2[a]	26.1[a]	26.6[a]	26.2[a]	25.1[b]	0.147	0.001
Mean daily CF intake(g/bird)	8.1[a]	7.9[a]	7.9[a]	8.0[a]	7.5[b]	0.064	0.002
Mean daily ME intake(kcal/bird)	431.2[ab]	433.2[ab]	438.6[a]	427.4[ab]	412.0[b]	3.018	0.024
Mean daily Ca intake(g/bird)	1.1[a]	1.1[a]	1.1[a]	1.1[a]	1.0[b]	0.015	0.001
Entire Experimental Period							
Mean daily DM intake (g/bird)	79.0[a]	78.9[a]	80.4[a]	78.5[ab]	75.8[b]	0.443	0.004
Mean total DM intake (g/bird)	4424.6[a]	4417.1[a]	4502.5[a]	4392.7[ab]	4245.8[b]	24.780	0.005
Mean daily CP intake(g/bird)	18.4[a]	18.4[a]	18.6[a]	18.3[a]	17.6[b]	0.099	0.002
Mean daily CF intake(g/bird)	5.2[a]	5.0[a]	5.1[a]	5.0[a]	4.5[b]	0.070	0.001
Mean daily ME intake(kcal/bird)	296.2[a]	303.8[a]	299.5[a]	292.6[a]	283.9[a]	2.308	0.078
Mean daily Ca intake(g/bird)	0.8[b]	0.8[b]	0.9[a]	0.9[a]	0.7[c]	0.020	0.001

Means with a different superscript in a row are significantly different (P< 0.05);DM-Dry Matter; CP- Crud Protein; CF- Crude Fibre; ME-Metabolizable Energy; Ca-Calcium; g gram; SEM-Standard Error of the Mean;T1-0%DBRCM+100%SBM Roasted; T2-20% DBRCM +80%SBM Roasted; T3-40%DBRCM+60%SBM Roasted; T4-60% DBRCM + 40% SBM Roasted; T5-80% DBRCM+20%SBM Roasted

Table 5. Body weight change of SASSO C44 broiler chicks in starter (1-28 days), finisher phases (29-56) and entire experiment (1-56 days) birds fed different level of dried blood rumen content mixture as a replacement for soybean meal

Parameters	Experimental Diets					SEM	P-value
	T1	T2	T3	T4	T5		
Starter Phase							
Initial bodyweight(g)	41.5[a]	41.2[a]	41.3[a]	41.0[a]	41.3[a]	0.406	0.998
Mean final body weight(g)	772.4[a]	768.8[ab]	729.4[ab]	753.8[ab]	696.3[b]	10.451	0.034
Mean daily weight gain(g/bird)	26.1[a]	26.0[ab]	24.6[ab]	25.5[ab]	23.4[b]	0.374	0.033
Mean total gain(g)	730.9[a]	727.7[ab]	688.1[ab]	712.8[ab]	655.1[b]	10.474	0.033
Finisher phase							
Initial bodyweight(g)	772.4[a]	768.8[ab]	729.4[ab]	753.8[ab]	696.3[b]	10.451	0.034
Mean final body weight(g)	1713.4[a]	1783.1[a]	1811.3[a]	1773.7[a]	1521.1[a]	41.612	0.203
Mean daily weight gain(g/bird)	33.6[a]	36.2[a]	38.6[a]	36.4[a]	29.5[a]	1.414	0.363
Mean total gain(g)	941.0[a]	1014.3[a]	1081.9[a]	1019.9[a]	824.8[a]	39.604	0.360
Entire Experimental Period							
Initial bodyweight(g)	41.5[a]	41.2[a]	41.3[a]	41.0[a]	41.3[a]	0.407	0.998
Mean final body weight(g)	1713.4[a]	1783.1[a]	1811.3[a]	1773.7[a]	1521.1[a]	41.613	0.203
Mean daily weight gain(g/bird)	29.9[a]	31.1[a]	31.6[a]	31.0[a]	26.4[a]	0.745	0.203
Mean total gain(g)	1671.9[a]	1741.9[a]	1770.0[a]	1732.6[a]	1479.9[a]	41.741	0.205
Mortality rate (%)	0.7[a]	0.0[a]	0.3[a]	0.7[a]	1.0[a]	0.133	0.212

Means with a different superscript in a row are significantly different (P< 0.05); g- gram; T1-0%DBRCM+100%SBM Roasted; T2-20% DBRCM +80%SBM Roasted; T3-40%DBRCM + 60%SBM Roasted; T4-60% DBRCM + 40% SBM Roasted; T5-80% DBRCM+20%SBM Roasted; SEM-Standard Error of the Mean

Table 6. Feed and nutrient conversion ratio of broilers fed diets with different levels of DBRCM for SBM during the starter phase (1-28 days), finisher phase (29-56 days) and the entire experimental period (1-56 days).

Parameters	Experimental Diets					SEM	P-value
	T1	T2	T3	T4	T5		
Starter Phase							
Feed conversion ratio(g DMI I/g gain)	1.5[a]	1.5[a]	1.6[a]	1.5[a]	1.6[a]	0.020	0.153
Protein conversion ratio(g CPI/g gain)	0.40[a]	0.40[a]	0.40[a]	0.400[a]	0.43[a]	0.007	0.461
Energy conversion ratio(kcal MEI/g gain)	6.20[a]	6.73[a]	6.53[a]	6.23[a]	6.70[a]	0.142	0.708
Fiber conversion ratio(g CFI/g gain)	0.10[a]	0.10[a]	0.10[a]	0.10[a]	0.07[a]	0.007	0.461
Calcium conversion ratio(g Cal/g gain)	0.02[a]	0.02[a]	0.02[a]	0.02[a]	0.02	0.001	0.633
Finisher phase							
Feed conversion ratio(g DM I/g gain)	3.5[a]	3.4[a]	3.1[a]	3.2[a]	3.8[a]	0.125	0.513
Protein conversion ratio(g CPI/g gain)	0.77[a]	0.77[a]	0.70[a]	0.70[a]	0.83[a]	0.031	0.740
Energy conversion ratio(kcal MEI/g gain)	12.90[a]	12.57[a]	11.40[a]	11.77[a]	14.0[a]	0.435	0.418
Fiber conversion ratio(g CFI/g gain)	0.27[a]	0.23[a]	0.20[a]	0.20[a]	0.27[a]	0.013	0.309
Calcium conversion ratio(g Cal/g gain)	0.03[a]	0.03[a]	0.03[a]	0.03[a]	0.03[a]	0.001	0.865
Entire Experimental Period							
Feed conversion ratio(g DMI I/g gain)	2.7[a]	2.6[a]	2.6[a]	2.5[a]	2.9[a]	0.058	0.465
Protein conversion ratio(g CPI/g gain)	0.60[a]	0.60[a]	0.60[a]	0.60[a]	0.67[a]	0.013	0.371
Energy conversion ratio(kcal MEI/g gain)	9.97[a]	9.87[a]	9.50[a]	9.50[a]	10.73[a]	0.213	0.418
Fiber conversion ratio(g CFI/g gain)	0.20[a]	0.17[a]	0.20[a]	0.20[a]	0.20[a]	0.007	0.461
Calcium conversion ratio(g Cal/g gain)	0.03[a]	0.03[a]	0.03[a]	0.03[a]	0.03[a]	0.001	0.461

Means with a different superscript in a row are significantly different (P< 0.05);DMI-Dry Matter Intake; CPI- Crud Protein Intake; CFI-Crude FibreIntake; MEI-Metabolizable Energy Intake; Cal-Calcium Intake; g-gram; T1-0% DBRCM +100%SBM Roasted; T2-20% DBRCM +80%SBM Roasted; T3-40%DBRCM+60%SBM Roasted; T4-60% DBRCM + 40% SBM Roasted; T5-80% DBRCM+20%SBM Roasted ; SEM-Standard Error of the Mean

Body weight change during the finisher phase

The body weight change of birds during the finisher phase is presented in Table 5. The mean daily weight gain of birds were 33.6g, 36.2g, 38.6g, 36.4g and 29.5g/bird/day for T1, T2, T3, T4 and T5, respectively. Statistically the mean daily weight gain had not shown a significant difference (p>0.05) among the treatment groups. There was no statistical marked difference (p>0.05) in final body weight and mean total body weight gain among treatment groups. However, numerically birds fed at 80%DBRCM (T5) almost had the lowest body weight and body weight gain among other treatment groups

Body weight change during the entire experiment

The body weight change and mortality rate of birds is presented in Table 5. The mean daily weight gain of birds fed five dietary treatment groups were 29.9g, 31.1g, 31.6g, 31.0g and 26.4g /bird/day. There was a similar (P>0.05) daily body weight gain of birds in each treatment groups, and there was no a statistical significant difference (P>0.05) in final body weight, total body weight gain and mortality rate among the treatment groups. However, numerically birds fed at 80%DBRCM (T5) almost had the lowest body weight and body weight gain among other treatment groups in this entire experimental period

Feed and nutrient conversion ratio
The feed and nutrient conversion ratio of SASOO C44 broiler chicks fed different levels of dried blood rumen content mixture as a replacement of soybean meal is presented in Table 6. There was a similar (p>0.05) feed and nutrient conversion ratio among the treatment groups in starter phase, finisher phase and the entire experimental growth period.

Discussion

The chemical composition of dried blood rumen content mixture (DBRCM)
The chemical composition of DBRCM was 93.1% DM, 36.93% CP, 15.75% CF, 7.5%MM, 1.48%EE, 31.64% NFE, 2328.5kcal ME/Kg DM and 1.43% Ca. The DM content of the feed was similar to the report of Odunsi, (2003), 94% DM, Onu et al., (2011), 92.86% DM and Togun et al., (2009),94.8%DM. The crude protein content of DBRCM was 36.93%, this was confirmed by the report of Togun et al., (2009) who noted that 37.63%, and nearly similar with the report of Dairo et al., (2005), 33.81% and Adenui and Balogun, (2003), 31.42%. However, the result was incomparable with the report of Onu et al., (2011), Olukayode et al., (2008) and Odunsi, (2003) who reported that the CP content of the feed was 45.35%, 47%, and 46.1%, respectively.
The CF content of the feed was 15.75%, which was nearly comparable with Adenui and Balogun, (2003) 18.71% and incomparable with the report of Onu et al., (2011) 8.81%, Odunsi (2003) 6.38%, Togun et al., (2009) 9% and Olukayode et al., (2008) 9.59%. The mineral matter of the feed was similar with the report of Togun et al., (2009) 7.5%. However, it was lower than from the report of Onu et al., (2011) 15.42%, Odunsi, (2003) 23.4% and Olukayode et al., (2008) 11.6%.
The EE of the feed was 1.48% which is nearly comparable with the report of Odunsi, (2003) 2.13%, higher than the report of Adenui and Balogun, (2003) 0.88% and lower than Olukayode et al., (2008) 6.55% and Onu et al., (2011) 4.10%. The energy content of the feed (2328.5kcal ME/Kg DM) was nearly in line with the report of Onu et al., (2011) 2599.49 kcal ME /kg DM and Adenui and Balogun, (2003) 2686 Kcal ME /kgDM, however the result was disagree with the report of Olukayode et al., (2008). The chemical composition of the feed was different with the report of some authors. This difference might be the feed ingredients eaten by the animal, the gap between the feed eaten and the animal's slaughter, the microflora of the gut and the method of feed processing. When the animals fed dry grasses, straws (teff, barley, wheat etc), stovers (maize, sorghum) and energy concentrates might have lower CP content and higher metabolizable energy whereas animals feed leguminous plants and protein concentrates might have higher crude protein and low energy content. Even if the presence and the absence of fasting before slaughtering my affect the nutrient composition of the feed stuff. When the feed is waited in the gut without any degradable by micro flora affects the nutritional content. The rumen contains one of the most varied and dense microbial populations in nature (McDonald et al, 2002) such as the phycomycetous fungi, protozoa, bacteria and others that are involved in this process (Mohammed et al., 2008). Microbes in the rumen convert nutrients such as cellulose and Non-Protein Nitrogen (NPN) into microbial proteins such that the rumen acts as a natural continuous system for the production of single cell proteins (Javanovic and Cuperloric, 1977). Hungate (1966) revealed that the microbes of the rumen are able to synthesis beta-glucanases, which are needed for the breakdown of cellulose, hemicelluloses and phenolic polymers. Those authors reported that the processing of the feed was done by mixing of a 1:1 ratio freshly collected blood and wet rumen content in the same container, and then boiled, dried and analysed to utilise for feed ingredient.

Dry matter intake (DMI) of birds during the experimental period
Birds fed on five dietary treatment groups during the starter phase, had not shown a marked statistically difference (P>0.05) in daily DMI among the treatment groups. However in the total DMI of birds fed on T1 (0% DBRCM) had the highest (P<0.05) and on T5 (80% DBRCM) the lowest (P<0.05) total dry matter intake. In the finisher phases, birds fed on T5 (80% DBRCM) had the lowest (P<0.05) daily and total DMI compared with other treatment groups. In the whole entire experimental period of growth, birds fed on T5 (80% DBRM) had the lowest daily DMI (p<0.05) compared with T1 (0% DBRCM), T2 (20% DBRCM) and T3 (40% DBRCM).
The total DMI of birds fed on T5 (80% DBRCM) had shown the least TDMI (P<0.05) compared with T1 (0% DBRCM), T2 (20% DBRCM), and T3 (% DBRCM). The result is in line with the finding of Adenui and Balogun (2003) who reported that there was no significantly different (P>0.05) in dry matter intake by pullets on the 10% BBRCM diet. However, this result is not in agreement with the report of Onu et al., (2011) who reported that the feed intake of broilers at finisher phases fed diet containing 0% BBRCM was significantly (P< 0.05) higher than those fed a diet containing BBRCM (Onu et al, 2011).

The result is not in line with the report of Olukayode et al., (2008) who noted that up to 10% of sun dried rumen blood had shown the higher feed intake compared with 15%SDRBM. Esonu et al., (2011) also reported that bird fed fermented bovine blood and rumen digesta (FBBRD) on finisher phases of growth, the highest feed intake values was recorded up to 10% inclusion level.

The result also disagrees with the finding of Adenui and Balogun, (2003) who indicated that, grower pullets fed with different levels of BBRCM diets; a higher (P<0.05) feed intake was observed in the birds fed on the 20% BBRCM diet. The disagreement continued with the report of Shim et al., (1989) and Pond (1989) who reported that feed intake was higher on fibrous diets, which could have caused the very high feed intake by the pullets on 20% BBRCM diet. When the inclusion level was increased at 80% DBRCM, the DMI is reduced. This is probably due to increasing fibrousness of the diets as the inclusion level of DBCRM was increased. According to Bolarinwa (1998) when the increased inclusion level of DBRCM may increase the fiber content, fiber limits feed utilization in poultry production. Onu et al., (2011) reported that the reduced intake of the birds on high level increment of DBRCM diets could be attributed to depressed appetite resulting from the unpleasant smell of the diets.

Odunsi (2003) also reported that the high level inclusion of blood meal and / or rumen content resulted unpleasant odour and make it less palatable to birds causing a depression in consumption. The same author stated that, the diets became darker in colour and the odor more accentuated with an increase in BBRDM. The combination of these two factors will negatively influence palatability resulting in low consumption.

Nutrient intake of birds fed with different levels of DBRCM

The CPI was ranged from 17.6-18.6 g/bird /day for whole entire period of the experiment. This result was in agreement with the report of Thirumalesh et al., (2012) who reported that the average daily CP intake was 19.9g/bird/day. The obtained result also nearly similar with the report of Kiros (2011) who noted that the CPI of birds 14.2-18.4g for the whole period of the experiment. The result was disagree with the report of Das et al.,(2010) who reported that the average CPI ranged from 13.5-13.8gram/ bird/ day. Birds fed on 20% DBRCM (T2) had a significant difference (p<0.05) in daily CP intake compared with birds fed on 80% DBRCM (T5) in the starter phase. Birds fed on 80%DBRCM (T5) had the lowest (P<0.05) CPI among other treatment groups both in the finisher phase and the entire experimental period.

The crude fiber intake ranged from 4.5-5.2 for the whole experimental period. The result was confirmed by the report of Kiros (2011) who noted that the daily CFI of broiler ranged 4.34-6.2 during the whole experimental period. The result was in line with the report of Thirumalesh et al., (2012) who reported that the CF intake of the whole period ranged from 4.4-5.3g/b/day. Different result was observed from the report of Das et al.(2010) who indicated that the CF intake ranged 2.56-2.61gram/bird/day. The CF intake of birds on 80%DBRCM (T5) was the lowest (P<0.05) daily intake compared with other treatment groups.

The Metabolizable energy intake ranged 283.9-303.8kcal in the entire experimental period. The same result was observed by Thirumalesh, et al., (2012) who noted that the average kcal intake was 306.6 and 307.7kcal in summer and winter season, respectively in the whole period of the experiment. The result is not in line with the report of Kiros (2011) who reported that the ME intake 212.5-276.7kcal. There was no a marked statistical difference in Metabolizable energy intake when birds fed on 0%, 20%, 40%, 60% and 80% of DBRCM.

The mean daily Calcium intake was 0.7- 0.9g/bird/day in the entire experimental period, however significantly the lowest (P<0.05) Ca intake was observed birds fed on 80% DBRCM (T5). This result indicates that, the substitution of DBRCM at 80% for soybean meal reduced the dry matter and nutrient intake.

When birds fed the lowest dry matter intake, accordingly the nutrient intake of the bird was reduced. Onu et al (2011) reported that the dry matter and nutrient intake decreased with increased the level of BBRCM. This is probably due to increasing fibrousness of the diets as the inclusion level of DBRCM was increased since fiber limits feed utilization in poultry production (Onifade, 1993; Bolarinwa, 1998). According to the report of Esonu et al., (2005), the crude fibre activates the intestine and more occurrences of peristaltic movement and enzyme production resulting in efficient digestion of nutrients. However, the inclusion level was becoming at large, the intake was reduced.

The higher crude fibre content of the test material which tends to increase the total fiibre content of the diets and dilute other nutrients, which may probably have interrupted intake, the digestibility and effective utilization of the nutrients in the diets (Esonu et al, 2011).

Body weight change

In this study the total body weight ranged from 1521.1- 1811.3gram in 56 experimental periods. The result was not confirmed by SASSO C44 broiler breeder (http://www.sasso.fr/best-chicken-breeds-alternative-growth-for-free-range-poultry_breeding.html,retrived on 20/03/ 2016) who reported that the average body weight of Sasso C44 broiler birds ranged from 2200-2700g in in 56 days of age. The result is not also in line with the reported of Henn et al., (2014) who noted that the average body weight of Sasso C44 broiler birds was 2123.5g in 49 experimental days of age. Birds fed on 80% DBRCM (T5) has shown statistically the lowest

(P<0.05) daily and total body weight gain among other dietary treatments in the starter phase of growth. In finisher phase and the whole experimental period, the mean daily and total body weight gain had not shown a statistical significant difference (P>0.05) among the treatment groups. However, numerically the substation of DBRCM at 40% (T3) had shown the highest average daily body weight gain 38.6g and 31.6 g for finisher phase and entire experimental period, respectively; while birds fed on 80%(T5) DBRCM shown the lowest mean daily body weight gain 29.5g and 26.4g for finisher and the whole entire period, respectively. Numerically the final body weight in the entire experimental period was the highest on 40% DBRC (T3), 1811.3 gram and the lowest on 80%DBRCM (T5), 1521.1 gm. Statistically there was not a significant different (p>0.05) observed among treatment groups in the final body weight of birds in the entire experimental period. Numerically, the total and daily body weight gain and the final body weight of a bird was linearly increased when birds fed on 0%, 20%, 40% DBRCM and then declined on 60 % DBRCM (T4) and 80% DBRCM (T5). The result confirmed the report of Olukayode et al, (2008) who noted that final body weight and body weight gain were superior (p < 0.05) for birds fed 10% SDRBM compared with all other diets in both the finisher phase and the entire period. The similar result was observed by Esonu et al, (2011) who reported that the body weight gain of the birds were numerically increased linearly up to 10% inclusion level of FBBRCM and then decreasing was observed. Statistically the same result was observed by Adenui and Balogun, (2003) who indicated that pullets fed different levels of BBRCM, there was no statistical different (P>O.05) in growth rates of birds as the BBRCM level of their diet increased. The result in lines with Emmanuel (1978) who concluded that whole rumen contents did not affect (P>0.05) growth when included in the diets of broiler from 1-21 days of age. Also similar result was reported by AFRIS (2010) who noted that the weight gain of broilers was not found (p>0.05) to be depressed when birds fed 10 to 15% dried rumen contents. The result is not disagree with the finding of Onu et al., (2011) who noted that body weight gain increased linearly (P < 0.05) with increase in the level of bovine blood rumen content meal of broilers. The improved weight gain of birds fed BBRCM diets could be attributed to higher protein content of the diets which were efficiently metabolized for growth (Onu et al., 2011). According to Esonu et al., (2004), chicks become difficult to utilize high fibre diets when the inclusion level of DBRCM is increased and adult birds utilize high fibre materials than chicks (Esonu et al., 2004). So that the finisher birds could tolerate DBRCM diets better than the chicks, because at this stage, they have a more developed gastro intestinal tract to handle the fibre contents of the diets (Esonu et al., 2004). Due to this reason, statistically similar (P>0.05) final body weight and body weight gain was observed in finisher and the entire experimental period up to 80% DBRCM inclusion level regardless of the numerical difference.

Feed and nutrient conversion ratio

Feed conversion ratio of the experimental chicks expressed as grams of feed consumed per unit body weight gain. Feed conversion ratio is considered as one of the leading quality parameter and its progress or development is generally associated with feed efficiency in poultry production. The feed and nutrient conversion ratio of birds fed the five dietary treatment groups had not shown a statistical significant difference (P>0.05) in starter, finisher phase and the entire experimental period.

Numerically birds fed at 80% DBRCM (T5) had shown the lowest feed conversion ratio in both growth periods. This result confirmed the report of Esonu et al, (2011) who noted that there was no significant difference (p>0.05) among the groups fed a diet containing different levels of feremented bovine blood rumen digesta (FBBRD) on feed conversion ratio in broiler chicks.

The same result was observed from the report of Dairo et al., (2005) who indicated that there was no a significant difference (P>0.05) in FCR in rabbits fed different levels of bovine blood rumen content mixture. The result in lines with Emmanuel (1978) who concluded that whole rumen contents did not affect (P>0.05) feed conversion when included in the diets of broiler from 1-21 days of age. Okorie (2005) reported similar results that dried pulverized rumen contents were no significant differences in FCR among birds that were given these diets. Also similar result was reported by AFRIS (2010) who noted that the FCR of broilers was not found (p>0.05) to be depressed when 10 to 15% dried rumen contents were fed.

The different result was observed by the report of Onu et al, (2011) who reported that a significant improvement (P<0.05) was seen in feed conversion ratio of birds as the level of BBRCM inclusion in the diets increased in finisher phases. The finding also not confirmed the reports of Adeniji and Balogun (2002) and Odunsi (2003) who reported that the significant difference (P<0.05) was observed in FCR of birds fed different levels of blood rumen content.

Numerically birds fed at 80% DBRCM (T5) had shown the lowest feed conversion ratio in both growth periods. According to Pond et al., (1989) high fibre diets reduce feed/gain ration, probably because it is the grower phase where growth rate tends to be reduced. However in this study the inclusion of DBRCM up to 80% for the replacement of SBM in broiler diets didn't affect the feed and nutrient conversion ratio in both growth phases.

Conclusion

Based on this study it could be concluded that in both phases of growth, the dry matter and nutrient intake was similar up to 60% substitution level and then reduced when it reaches at 80%inclusion level. The body weight gain was not affected up to 60% inclusion level in starter phase. However the substitution of DBRCM up to 80% inclusion level did not affect the daily and final body weight gain in finisher phase and the entire experimental period of growth. At 80% substitution level of DBRCM in broiler ration didn't affect the feed and nutrient conversion ratio and mortality rate of birds in both growth periods.

Therefore dried blood rumen content mixture at 60% substitution level can replace soybean meal without any deleterious effect in dry matter and nutrient intake, body weight gain, and feed and nutrient conversion ratio up to 28 days of growth period; and up to 80% DBRCM substitution level can replace the soybean meal in finisher and entire experimental growth period of birds without affecting body weight change, feed and nutrient conversion ratio and mortality rate.

Acknowledgment

The author is especially acknowledged to Debre Markos University for its permission and financial support to study my PhD. Besides, I would like to thank College of Veterinary Medicine and Agriculture, Addis Ababa University for providing me with a good environment and facilitates to complete this PhD program.

References

1) A.O.A.C (Association of Official Analytical Chemists) (2000). Official Methods of Analysis. 13th Edition, Washington D.C.America.

2) Adeniji A.A. and Balogun O.O. (2002). Utilization of Flavour Treated Blood-Rumen Content Mixture In The Diet of Laying Hens. Nigeria Journal Animal Production 29(1): 34-39

3) Adeniji A. A. and Jimoh A. (2007). Effects of Replacing Maize with Enzyme- Supplemented Bovine Rumen Content in the Diets of Pullet Chicks. International Journal of Poultry Science 6 (11): 814-817

4) Adenui A. A. & Balogun O. O. (2003). Influence of Bovine Blood-Rumen Content Meal In The Diets of Growing Pullets on Their Subsequent Laying Performance. Department of Animal Production, University of florin, Nigeria, Ghana journal of Agricultural sciences 6, 47-51.

5) AFRIS (Animal Feed Resources Information System) (2010). file://C:Documents and Setting/ADMIN/My Document Retrieved 26/4/2010.

6) Bisrat G.U. (2013). Defect Assessment of Ethiopian Hide and Skin: The Case of Tanneries in Addis Ababa and Modjo, Ethiopia, Ethiopian Leather Industry Development Institute (LIDI), Addis Ababa, Ethiopia . Global Veterinaria 11 (4): 395-398

7) CSA (Central Statistical Agency) (2013). Livestock Statistics. CSA, Federal Democratic Republic of Ethiopia, Addis Ababa, Ethiopia

8) Bolarinwa B.B. (1998). Evaluation and Optimum Use of Fibrous Ingredients In The Diets Of Broilers. Ph.D.Thesis, University of Ibadan, Ibadan, Nigeria.

9) Dairo F.A.S. (2005). Assessment of Rumen Content on the Haematological Parameters Of Growing Rabbits: Proc. of 10th Annual Conference of Animal Science Association of Nigeria (ASAN), Sept. 12-15. University of Ado Ekiti, Nigeria. Pp. 301-302.

10) Das T.K., Mondal M.K., Biswas P., Bairagi B. and Samanta C.C. (2010). Influence of Level of Dietary Inorganic and Organic Copper and Energy Level on the Performance and Nutrient Utilization of Broiler Chickens. Asian-Australasian Journal of Animal Sciences 23(1): 82-89

11) Dominguez-Bello M.G., Michelangeli J., Ruis M.C., Garcia A., Rodriguez E. (1994). Ecology of The Folivorous Hoatzin (Opisthocomus hoazin) On The Venezuelan Plains. The Auk 111 (3): 643-65

12) Downes T.E.H., Nourse L.D., Siebrits F.K. and Hastings J.W. (1987). The relative nutritive value of irradiated spray-dried blood powder and heat-sterilized blood meal as measured in combination with whey protein. South African journal of Animal Science 17(2):55-58

13) Emmanuel B. (1978). Effect of rumen content of fraction thereon in performance of broiler birds. Journal of Poultry Science, 19: Pp. 13-16.

14) Esonu B. O., Azubuike J. C., Emenalom O. O., Etuk E. B., Okoli I. C., Ukwu H. O. and Nneji C. S. (2004). Effect Of Enzyme Supplementation On The Performance Of Broiler Finisher Fed Microdesmis puberula Leaf Meal. International journal of poultry sciences 3: 112-114.

15) Esonu B.O., Izukanne K.O. and Inyang O. . (2005). Evaluation Of Cellulolytic Enzyme Supplementation On Production Indices And Nutrient Utilization Of Laying Hen Fed Soyabean Hull Based Diets. International Journal of Poultry Science 4(3): 114-120.

16) Esonu B.O., Azubuike J.C., Udedibie A., Emenalom O.O., Iwuji T.C and Odoemenam V. (2011). Evaluation of the Nutritive Value of Mixture of Fermented Bovine Blood and Rumen Digesta for Broiler Finisher Journal of Natural Sciences Research 1(4): 65-71.

17) Henn JD., Bockor L.,Ribeiro AML., Coldebella A.and Kessler A. M. (2014). Growth and Deposition of Body Components of Intermediate and High Performance Broilers. Brazilian Journal of Poultry Science, 16 (3): 319-328

18) Hungate R.E. (1966). The rumen and its microbes. Academic Press, New York and London. Pp 533

19) Javanovic M. and Cuperlovic M. (1977). Nutritive value of rumen contents for monogastric animals. Animal and Feed Science Technology 2: 351-360.

20) Kiros A. (2011). Evaluation of Sugar Syrup as a Partial Substitute for Maize in Broilers' Ration. MSc thesis Submitted to the School of Graduate Studies in Haramaya University, Ethiopia. pp 24-32

21) Liu D.C. (2009). Better Utilization of By-Products from the Meat Industry. Department of Animal Science. National Chung-Hising University Taichung Taiwan Roc.www.agnet.org/library/teb/515/eb/515.pdf Retrieved on 4/11/2009.

22) McDonald P., Edwards R.A., Greenhalgh J.F.D. and Morgan C.A. (2002). Animal Nutrition India 6th ed, Pearson Education Plc. Ltd Publishers, 2002.

23) Mohammed G., Igwebuike J.U., Ubosi C.O. and Alade N.K. (2008). Comparative study of the nutrient composition, Amino acid profile and microbial Assay of fresh and dry cattle, camel, sheep, and goat, rumen contents. Proceedings of 13th annual conference of animal science association of Nigeria (ASAN) Sep 15-19, 2008. p-518-520

24) NRC (National Research Council) (1994). Nutrient Requirements of Poultry. 9th Revised Edition. National Academic Press, Washinton DC.

25) Odunsi A.A. (2003). Blend of Bovine Blood and Rumen Digesta as a Replacement for Fishmeal and Groundnut Cake in Layer Diets. International Journal of Poultry Science 2 (1): 58-61

26) Okorie K.C. (2005). The effects of dried pulverized rumen content on the performance, carcass and organ characteristics of broiler finisher. Animal Production and Resource Advances 2: 96-100

27) Olukayode M., Babafunso S. and Segun A. (2008). Conversion of Abattoir Wastes Into Livestock Feed: Chemical Composition of Sun-Dried Rumen Content Blood Meal And Its Effect on Performance of Broiler Chickens, Conference on International Research on Food Security, Natural Resource Management and Rural Development University of Hohenheim, Nigeria.

28) Onifade A. A. (1993). Comparative utilization of three dietary fibres in broiler chickens. Ph.D. Thesis, University of Ibadan, Ibadan, Nigeria.

29) Onu P.N., Otuma M.O., Odukwe C.A. and Aniebo A.O. (2011). Effects of Different Levels of Bovine Blood / Rumen Content Mixture on Productive Performance, Carcass Characteristics and Economics of Production of Finisher Broilers. International Journal of Food, Agriculture and Veterinary Sciences 1 (1): 10-16.

30) Pond W. G., DicksonJ. S. & Itacheck, W.M. (1989). Comparative Response of Swine and Rats to High Fibre or High Protein Diets. Journal of Animal Science 67: 716- 723.

31) SAS (Statistical Analysis Systems, Version 9.2), (2008). Statistical Analysis Systems for mixed models. SAS Institute Inc, Cary, NC, USA.

32) SASSO C44 broiler Breeds: http://www.sasso.fr/best-chicken-breeds-alternative-growth-for-free-range-poultry-breeding.html, retrieved on 20/03/ 2016).

33) Shim K. F., Chen T. W., Teo L. H. & Khin M. M. (1989). Utilization of Wet Spent Grains by Ducks. Nutrition Reports International 40: 261-266.

34) SPSS (2012). Statistical Package for Social Science, SPSS 20 for Windows. SPSS Inc. Chicago, Illinois

35) Thirumalesh T., Ramesh B.K. and Suresh B.N. (2012). Influence Of Season on Nutrient Intake And Performance of broilers In Arid Region Of Karnataka. Indian Journal of Animal Resources, 46 (1): 78 – 81

36) Togun V.A., Farinu G.O., Ojebiyi O.O., Awotunde A.I. (2009). Effect Of Replacing Maize With A Mixture of Rumen Content And Blood Meal on the Performances of Growing Rabbits: Initial Study With Mash Feed. World Rabbit Science 17: 21-26

37) Wiseman J. (1987). Feeding of Non-Ruminant Livestock. Butterworth and C.Ltd. pp. 370

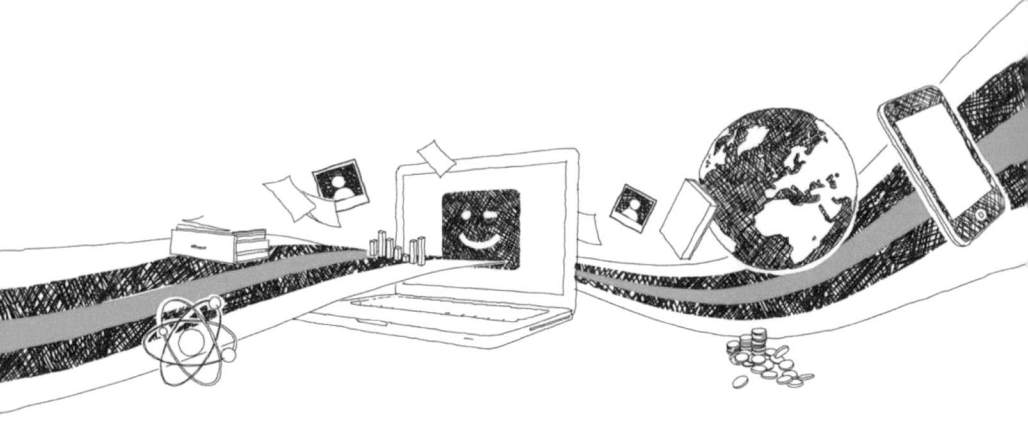
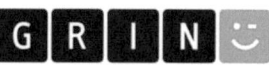